I Feel Like Me Again!

Offering Hope To Women With Special Healthcare Needs

I Feel Like Me Again!

The Story of Women's Health Boutique

By
Nancy Arnold

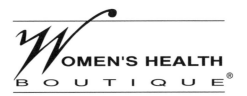

Developed by Women, For Women,
To Meet Women's Unique Health-Related Needs

I FEEL LIKE ME AGAIN!

Library of Congress Cataloging-in-Publication Data:

Arnold, Nancy, 1946-
I Feel Like Me Again!/ Nancy Arnold.
   p.   cm.
ISBN 0-9645102-2-7
1. Success in business—United States—Case studies. 2. Women's Health Boutique—History.   3. Arnold, Nancy, 1946-
   . I. Title.
98-74345

2 3 4 5 9 MVP 9 8 7 6 5 4 3 2

Printed in the United States of America

2nd Edition   1999

Dedicated to the memory of
Billie Marie Dortch

Her life was an example…
Her illness was a challenge…
Her death led to inspiration…

Contents

Message from Vicki Dortch Jones

Founder
Women's Health Boutique Franchise System, Inc.

When our mother, Billie Dortch, was diagnosed with terminal cancer in 1986 at the age of 56, none of us knew then that her struggle would inspire the creation of Women's Health Boutique. We were just grateful to get through each day, each new challenge. Our mother and her well being was our world then.

With formidable strength and perseverance, she continued to work every day, ministering to and touching the lives of others. For well over a year, we watched, as little by little, she was robbed of her dignity.

My sister Seleta and I were frustrated, wanting so much to make her daily life easier and help restore her dignity. This was really brought home to us when our mother, this wonderful, dignified lady, chose to "go bald" rather than wear the ill-fitting wig that irritated her skin and looked nothing like her own hair.

It was only after she died that we were amazed to find so many products that could have helped her, could have made her life more comfortable, and that could have restored her dignity.

This terrible time gave me the passion to explore and develop the full realm of women's health.

I was appalled to discover the inadequacies in women's health care. This despite the fact that two-thirds of all surgeries in the United States are performed on women, and two out of every three health care dollars are spent by women!

I was shocked to learn that breast cancer is the leading cause of death for women between the ages of 35 and 54, striking down over 40,000 women a year. My husband's mother died of breast cancer when she was only 45 years old! But I was encouraged by knowing that more and more women survive this awful disease, thanks to early detection and improved treatment.

These women, these survivors, needed somewhere to go where their dignity could be restored following this terrible assault. They needed to know they can feel pretty again, that they can feel desirable again, that they can feel normal again.

Women's Health Boutique became that somewhere. Now a woman with special healthcare needs can find what she needs, all in one beautiful, special place to shop.

A woman is still a woman, whether she's lost a breast or her hair, has lymphedema or varicose veins, or is experiencing a difficult pregnancy. She has the same needs for femininity, sensitivity and dignity.

This book is about real women who have found hope and dignity and respect at Women's Health Boutiques across the country. These women could be your own mother, sister, daughter, wife, friend...or you.

Our mother should have had access to the myriad products out there that would have made her battle with cancer easier. Every woman should have a place to go where her special healthcare needs can be met.

Women's Health Boutique is our mother's legacy to you...to us...to women everywhere. I know she would be pleased.

Acknowledgements

Vicki Dortch Jones

Her compassion inspired her and her enthusiasm carried her as she sought to build a place where women with special healthcare needs could have those needs met with respect and sensitivity…and maybe just a hug or two.

Seleta Dortch Lovell

Seleta worked by her mother's side, learning the home medical equipment business her mother had built. As Women's Health Boutique developed, Seleta provided strong business management that led to a successful acquisition by ICED. Although no longer active in WHB, her contributions continue to have an impact.

Bud Hadfield

With his unique vision he was able to see how Women's Health Boutique could grow and become a household name in the ever-expanding healthcare arena. His decades of experience in franchising, coupled with his own perseverance and success, provided the inspiration and direction for developing WHB.

Steve Hammerstein

His calm guidance and natural leadership skills, combined with a true sense of respect for women, mean so much as Women's Health Boutique moves toward becoming a household name in communities across the country.

And finally…to women everywhere who deserve the best products and services available to help them meet any healthcare crisis with dignity. Women's Health Boutique's mission statement is simple: to meet women's special needs and make a positive difference in the way women look and feel about themselves.

A Personal Note from the Author

Women's Health Boutique is, without a doubt, one of the most exciting concepts to hit the healthcare industry. Wow! A business in a boutique setting focusing exclusively on women's health! When I first heard of it, I thought "finally, someone has listened to us and understands what we need."

The more I learned, the more excited I became. As a woman, I know firsthand the frustrations of not being able to find a product, a service, or just information, about some strictly female issue. But no more! Women's Health Boutique is there for me, my mother, my daughter, my sisters and my friends.

It has been a privilege for me to tell the story of Women's Health Boutique. As you read about the many health issues all of us women will face at some time in our lives, I know you'll feel the relief I felt to learn there are solutions.

When you read the stories of several women who have been helped at the boutiques, you'll probably shed a tear, as much for them as for yourself or others you know who could have found help if only there had been a place like this.

Now there is a place, and it's long overdue. Come with me as I tell you the story of Women's Health Boutique.

Nancy Arnold

Section

1

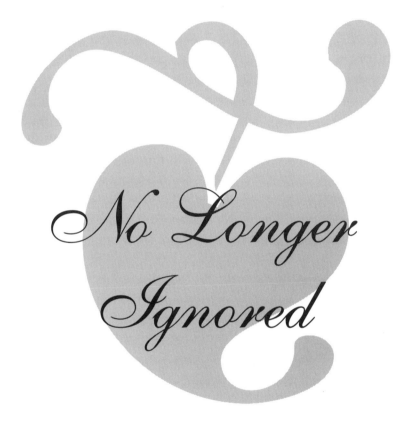

No Longer Ignored

*W*omen's health issues have only been specifically addressed in the last decade or so. Even today, clinical trials are primarily conducted on men because scientists fear damage to the reproductive organs of female participants, according to Dr. Sandra Hoffman, assistant professor of medicine and coordinator of the MSU/KCMS women's health curriculum.

Estrogen therapy, as common as chewing gum, was originally tested as a cholesterol-lowering agent for men, and has never really been extensively tested on women, says Dr. Hoffman.

Those involved with Women's Health Boutique are troubled by these and other statistics about women's health, and the largely unmet needs of the women involved. Consider these facts:

- ❦ Two-thirds of all surgeries in the United States are performed on women.
- ❦ Two out of every three health care dollars are spent by women.
- ❦ 140,000 women a year survive breast cancer and need products and services to help them resume their lives.
- ❦ An estimated 20 million women have some form of female pattern baldness or medically related hair loss, and they need everything from wigs and hairpieces to hats and turbans, plus the care products for those items.
- ❦ Over 75% of all pregnant women work into their third trimester and more products are being developed for those women every day.
- ❦ Over 70% of all new mothers choose to breastfeed and need education, breastfeeding supplies and support garments.
- ❦ Eight out of 10 women are wearing the wrong size bra and need the help of professional fitters for comfort and health.
- ❦ 8.5 million women of all ages suffer from some form of urinary incontinence and need help managing this condition.
- ❦ Skin care is a vital, yet overlooked concern for millions of women secondary to mastectomy, pre-and post-partum,

radiation treatment, chemotherapy, incontinence, diabetes and more.

New products are being developed daily to meet the unique health needs of today's woman. Women's health will easily be one of the strongest segments of the American economy well into the next century.

Women's Health Boutique has a unique retailing concept that is perfectly positioned to take full advantage of this rapidly expanding market.

As part of the ICED family of international franchises, this franchise is poised to provide a high level of attention to women's health issues and to a new segment of business opportunity.

Steve Hammerstein, President and CEO of ICED, says the franchising giant intends to expand the WHB Franchise System nationwide, in addition to the units already in operation. "Women's Health Boutique is a new and exciting concept in one of the fastest growing segments of our economy – the healthcare industry," stated Hammerstein.

He goes on to say, "The exciting thing about this wonderful alliance is that ours is the only system focusing exclusively on women's health, and ICED plans to grow quickly to secure this market."

According to Hammerstein, ICED also intends to continue its franchise expansion into healthcare by adding other health-related franchises to the family. He adds, "This alliance is an excellent business opportunity for us to successfully apply our franchise experience to yet another industry."

Hammerstein says all the resources of ICED are being utilized so that Women's Health Boutique becomes well-known, both in the medical world and to the women everywhere who need that one place where they can receive help coping with the health challenges that will come their way.

The Breast Cancer Wars... Surviving Can Be Hell, Too

*B*reast cancer. That diagnosis is given to over 180,000 women a year. Almost 140,000 of those women will survive this terrible disease and must somehow learn to live with the aftermath. They need to know they can live, really live. They need to know they can feel pretty again. They need to know they can feel desirable. They need to feel normal.

Women's Health Boutique is where they can begin that journey back to their former lives, where they can learn to feel like themselves again. And that journey can begin within hours of surgery.

In most cases, the time between diagnosis and surgery is only a few days. That leaves very little time for coherent thought, much less planning a future wardrobe. But the fact is, from the time the bandages are removed, wardrobe does become important.

Starting with getting dressed to leave the hospital, a woman discovers she now has a bra, and many others at home just like it, that just doesn't work anymore. Where once she had shape and balanced weight, she's now lopsided. What can she do? Where can she go? Who can help her?

Doctors and other health care professionals spend so much time dealing with the medical and clinical aspects of breast cancer that many times they aren't even aware of what products and services are out there for their patient. These products can make a real difference for a woman going home following the radical things that have happened to her body, and to her spirit.

Doctors are able to do what they need to do, but they are rarely able to address the 'what do I do with the rest of my life?' question that women face following breast cancer treatment.

In times past, women who needed a prosthesis went searching in either a clinical-looking medical supply store or an under-stocked drug store. They had to wander down the aisles, past the wheelchairs and colostomy bags, and finally find a shelf where a few prostheses were kept. The clerk, if there was one, was often a man. They received little guidance, were often improperly fitted

—if at all—and left the store feeling embarrassed and somehow ashamed.

Or even worse for a woman who has just suffered the utmost assault on her femininity, she had to go to a lingerie shop and stumble past racks of revealing garments she would never be able to wear again, to the back of the store, and still find herself poorly served.

Many women tell stories of just not wearing a prosthesis of any kind because of the frustrations of trying to find one that fit and a bra to accommodate it. They concede defeat, putting their pretty fitted dresses and shirts in the back of the closet.

For a woman who has had a breast removed, the issues she now faces involve more than vanity. The body is suddenly out of balance. Where once there was weight and mass on her chest to balance her frame, now there is nothing. The frame—the body—suffers. It becomes a health issue, not just a cosmetic issue.

Following breast cancer treatment, a woman may experience lymphedema, hair loss from radiation or chemotherapy, and skin care problems. She needs the correct breast prosthesis, a properly fitted bra, and perhaps wigs or head wraps. She desires stylish and pretty garments she can wear comfortably. And she wants emotional support to help her feel comfortable with her new, sometimes alien, body.

Lymphedema, for instance, can significantly affect up to 35% of mastectomy patients. This condition is caused when lymph nodes are removed during surgery. The flow of lymphatic fluid through the body is disrupted.

This results in swelling, usually in the upper arm, caused when the fluids collect in one area. After a woman has consulted with her doctor, she can come to Women's Health Boutique, where professionally trained staff members can help her explore products and methods for controlling this condition.

WHB began because of cancer. Founders Vicki D. Jones and Seleta Lovell experienced the frustrations of trying to find products and garments to ease their mother's daily life as she battled the disease. They discovered firsthand the trials of knowing those aids must be out there, but finding there was no one place to look.

Now there is. At Women's Health Boutique, a woman will find a wide variety of products designed to meet her special needs. For the woman who has just had breast surgery, there are camisoles, radiation garments and breast forms. She can choose bras and lingerie, wigs and turbans. To help her resume her life, there are swimwear and swim forms, partial forms and enhancers, compression garments and more.

Care of the skin immediately following mastectomy is very important because the skin of the chest has not healed sufficiently to allow the final prosthesis to be worn. The specialty skin care product line includes several uniquely designed for use on the healing tissue and to keep the skin soft and pliable.

For this transition period, WHB offers a 100% cotton post-surgical camisole designed specifically to provide maximum comfort and protection against the tender incision. This garment includes a foam prosthesis that will give shape and security following surgery until a woman can be properly fitted for a prosthesis and mastectomy bra. A woman may wear this garment home from the hospital. This gives her added confidence to face her family and friends.

Non-surgical Alternatives

Because of all the controversy over internal implants, more and more women are opting for external prostheses. For instance, there's a custom-made external breast reconstruction that can be worn continuously for four or five days. This product adheres to the chest wall with a Velcro®-like strip, and is comfortable even while sleeping or with bathing suits and lingerie, much to the delight of women who use them.

There's also an external prosthesis that adheres directly to the chest wall without the strips. Designed to be removed upon retiring, it is less expensive because there are no strips to purchase, but it is just as comfortable.

The cost for the custom-made prosthesis, at well under $3,000, is a very attractive alternative to surgical reconstruction at many times that cost. Because it is external, it is completely safe, and it provides a woman with a natural looking product that even matches her own skin tones.

Other prostheses may range from $30-$450, depending on their intended use. The certified fitters at WHB will help each woman choose the appropriate size and shape. Most of these prostheses are in stock and can be worn out of the boutique the same day they're fitted.

Regardless of which prosthesis is chosen, many insurance companies, even managed care companies, may pick up all or part of the costs for at least one prosthesis a year.

Hair Loss

While a woman can hide the loss of a breast, even without a prosthesis, she can't hide the fact that she has lost her hair. This loss is perhaps even more devastating to a woman than the loss of her breast. Each boutique offers dozens of wigs designed to fit over a snug-fitting cotton cap that holds the hairpiece in place.

The wigs look just like real hair, and come in various textures and colors. They can even be worn behind the ears, a nice surprise many women don't realize. These wigs can be trimmed and styled to a woman's own preference. Some women even buy two wigs, or experiment with the hair color they always wanted to try.

For the less daring woman, a wig can be custom made to match her own hair before treatment causes hair loss. Consultants will guide the woman in caring for her wig, and each boutique carries a complete inventory of wig care products.

There are occasions when a woman may not want to wear a full wig. For those times, there are fashionable turbans and wraps.

Some are made with fringes of hair in the back or bangs in the front to give the illusion of a full head of hair.

Inside Women's Health Boutique

When a woman enters a Women's Health Boutique, she is immediately aware that this is a place for her, where she will feel comfortable and important. Each of the boutiques is decorated in warm hues—rose, buttercup, soft teal. Flowery wallpaper, pretty draperies and elegant furniture adorn the rooms. Instead of countertops and cash registers, clients see beautiful tables and desks. Comfortable chairs and couches are spaced throughout the boutique. Music plays quietly in the background, and the fitting rooms are private and spacious.

One client said the ambiance is like someone's living room, where every visitor is treated like a family member or favorite guest. As one owner commented, a woman is reluctant to come into one of the stores, because that means she has a condition she doesn't want to have. But that feeling is quickly dispelled upon walking in as she absorbs the very comfortable environment.

WHB Staff Offers Care and Concern

The professional staff spends anywhere from five minutes to several hours helping individual clients, especially breast cancer survivors. They are there to help a woman in her first attempts to regain control of her life and her condition.

If a woman becomes anxious, they will stop and talk. They may even cry together. Good listening skills are important for all staff members, and while they don't counsel, they do understand the importance counseling plays in the healing process. They know where in the community they can refer their clients for professional counseling.

Sometimes the staff may find they are comforting husbands who just don't know what to say to their wives, or how to act around them.

Through it all, the boutique owners and staff really care about their clients. They are proud of the facilities and the impact they make in their communities, and in the lives of those they help.

Women's Health Boutique is truly a place where breast cancer survivors are made to feel special, and where dignity is free.

Hair Today. . . Gone Tomorrow

*C*rowning glory, shining locks, shimmering strands. A full head of hair is romanticized to the point that loss of hair is regarded as almost a moral failing.

Lady Godiva apparently had yards of cascading hair, enough to completely protect her modesty during that famous ride. Rapunzel, it is said, let down her rope-like tresses to her lover so he could climb to her tower prison and rescue her.

We're assaulted by television ads, magazine layouts and giant billboards that constantly remind us of the need for beautiful, thick, shining hair. Store shelves are lined with every conceivable hair care product, and hair salons are on every street corner. The relentless message is that to be a beautiful, sexy woman, we must have beautiful hair.

Yet an estimated 20 million women in the United States suddenly lose their hair for a variety of reasons. With it often goes their self-esteem and sometimes their very identity. Yes, hair is one of the more potent symbols of femininity and beauty. But does the loss of hair mean a woman is no longer desirable or attractive? The answer is a resounding *NO!*

Although loss of hair is a very public announcement that something is amiss, a woman can learn to turn stares into smiles just by the way she holds herself and in the way she interacts with others. In other words, her true personality, her playfulness, can emerge without the distraction of hair.

For some women, that's just not how she sees herself, and she can feel tremendously self-conscious and almost naked. When a woman feels this way, she can regain her self-confidence by finding creative new ways of covering her head.

What Causes Hair Loss?

Hair loss is caused by a variety of reasons. One of the more common is chemotherapy used in cancer treatment. This loss, if it occurs, is rapid and in large quantities. A woman may wake one morning to find clumps of hair on her pillow, and she is completely devastated.

The good news is that new hair will probably start growing in six months to a year, although it may initially be a different color or texture from the hair that was lost.

For abnormal hair loss, or alopecia (al-oh-PEE-sha), the many reasons may include:

- ❦ Physical stress: illness, surgery, anemia, rapid weight change
- ❦ Emotional stress: death of a family member, mental illness
- ❦ Medications: blood pressure or gout medications, high doses of Vitamin A, birth control pills
- ❦ Thyroid abnormalities
- ❦ Hormonal changes: pregnancy, menopause

Surgery, severe illness and emotional stress can cause hair loss because the body simply diverts its energies toward repair rather than production of hair. Some health conditions, such as anemia, low blood count or thyroid imbalance, may also contribute to chronic hair loss. These can be diagnosed with a simple blood test.

If a woman embarks on a stringent new diet, either on her own or through one of the many diet centers now in vogue, she may experience some hair loss. Because some of the structured diet plans include supplements high in Vitamin A, some women may see hair loss while on these programs.

Hormonal changes, either during pregnancy or menopause, or while taking birth control pills, can also cause hair loss. Regrowth usually occurs within three to six months following pregnancy or discontinuation of birth control pills.

But What Do I Do In The Meantime?

In almost all cases of abnormal hair loss, there may be a three month delay between the event and the beginning of hair loss. Then there may be another three month interval of regrowth.

That means there could be at least a six month period of partial or total hair loss.

Certainly it's not practical to remain at home for six months waiting for hair to grow back. So, it can be important for a woman to find new ways of covering her bare head. Coping with hair loss creatively can go a long way toward lifting the human spirit and improving self-image.

The WHB consultants are there to help any woman do just that—cope creatively. For the woman who's not quite ready to face the world "as is," there's a full selection of wigs, turbans and wraps. If a woman facing chemotherapy wants to, she can even have a wig custom-matched to her own hair color and texture before treatment begins.

This could be a time for a woman to express herself, let her playful nature emerge. Maybe a brunette always wanted to be a blonde or a redhead. A woman who's always worn her hair long can experiment with a pixie cut. With a wig, any look is possible.

Today's quality wigs are lighter and more versatile than ever before, and look and feel like real hair. They can be highlighted or trimmed to a woman's own preference. Women are pleasantly surprised to find they can even wear their new hair behind their ears or pulled back.

Turbans and scarf wraps are also available, providing yet another alternative to full wigs. Some turbans can be worn with a fringe of hair in the front or back. Special padding is available to give the illusion of hair underneath.

Many women prefer to wear some sort of head covering all the time, even while sleeping. The professionally trained consultants can help find the right combination of products to suit a particular lifestyle. They can also help determine whether insurance may cover all or part of the cost.

In the intimacy of the boutique, a woman can feel comfortable exploring her new look, and can get the necessary advice on the different types of headwear and how to care for it. In the case of irreversible hair loss, the informational material at the boutiques will be a valuable aid to her in learning how to deal with her new situation.

Yes, hair loss can be devastating to a woman, but it need not mean she must stay in the shadows or wear unattractive head coverings—not when Women's Health Boutique is there to help.

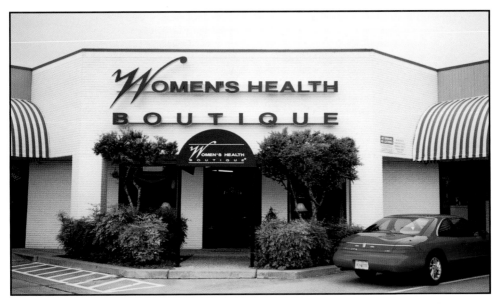

Women's Health Boutiques are open in many major metropolitan cities. They may be located near medical centers…

…or in nearby suburban shopping areas.

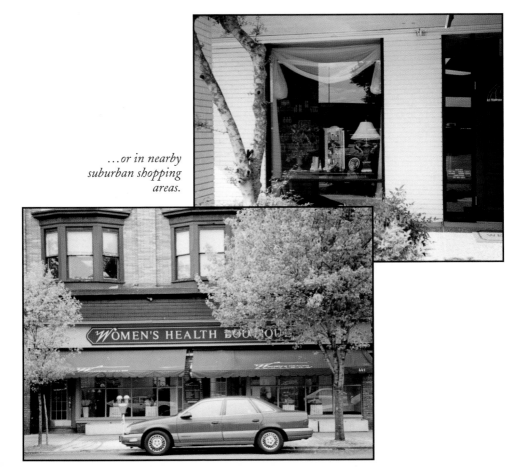

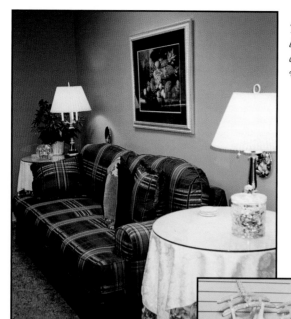

The warm ambience of the boutiques offer clients a calm, comfortable environment in which to face trying situations.

Certified fitters at Women's Health Boutique will assist women with special fitting needs, and help them select the most comfortable and attractive lingerie.

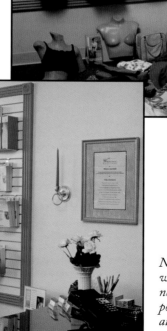

New and expectant mothers will find everything they need for their pre- and post-natal care and comfort at Women's Health Boutique.

The Educational Library at every boutique is filled with books, videos and audio tapes that women can check out and review in the privacy of their own home.

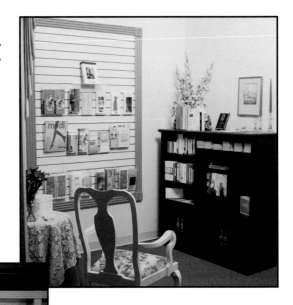

Women are delighted to find a full array of beautiful swimsuits specially designed to accommodate breast prostheses or enhancers.

At Women's Health Boutique every woman is special, and the consultants will spend as much time as needed to help meet her individual needs.

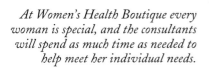

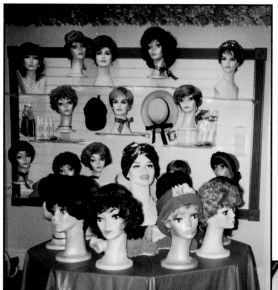

Each boutique offers a full selection of wigs, turbans, scarfs and wraps.

Each boutique offers professional wig styling by a licensed cosmetologist, as well as wig-care products to use at home.

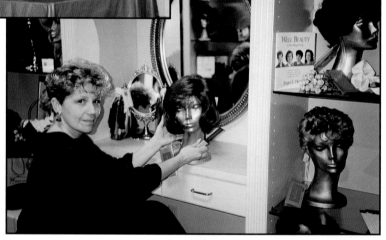

Speciality skin care products are available for those with pre-and post-partum needs; following mastectomy, radiation treatment and chemotherapy; and for those experiencing incontinence, diabetes and more.

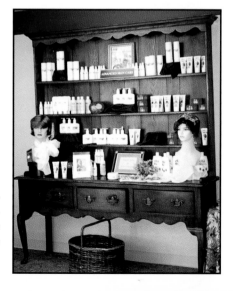

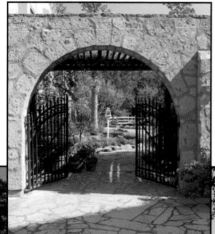

Tall iron gates on the grounds of ICED headquarters open onto a courtyard of flowers, filled with the soft music of a fountain.

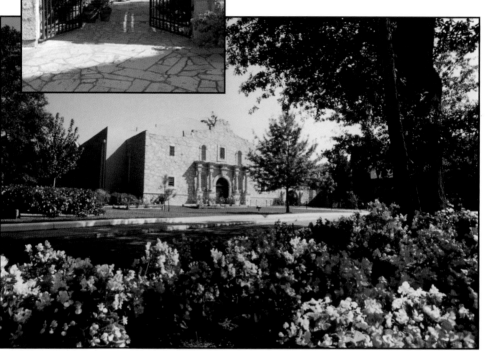

The Alamo occupies a special place in the hearts of all who believe that every man should walk proud and free. As our training facility, the Alamo at Northwest Forest fulfills this glorious tradition.

Inside the Alamo, a spacious atrium serves as a place for seminars, meetings, weddings and banquets. Upstairs rooms are named for Texas heroes.

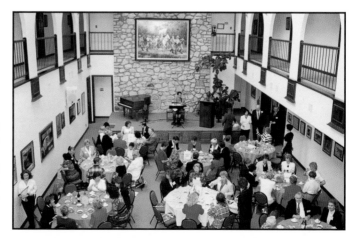

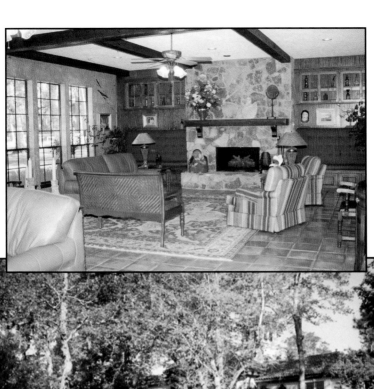

The lounge at La Hacienda is the perfect place to relax, or even to indulge in the most civilized of customs, la siesta.

La Hacienda, with its red tile roof and ornate balconies, evokes the timeless spell of Old Mexico. Lodging and meeting rooms are designed to welcome guests. "Mi casa es su casa."

The cloistered courtyard of La Hacienda is a place where time stands still.

Sturdy log buildings in a woodland setting add a frontier note. The "Log Inn," with its spotless kitchen, is our cafeteria.

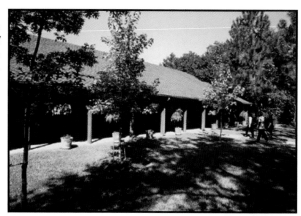

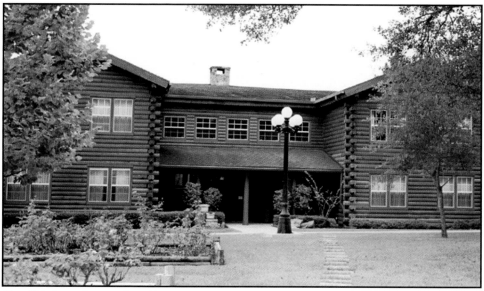

"Inn I" is home for new franchise owners, who come to us from around the world for their initial training.

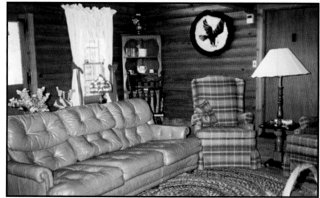

The lounge at "Inn I" is a gathering place for students occupying the ten comfortable apartments. Nothing has been overlooked.

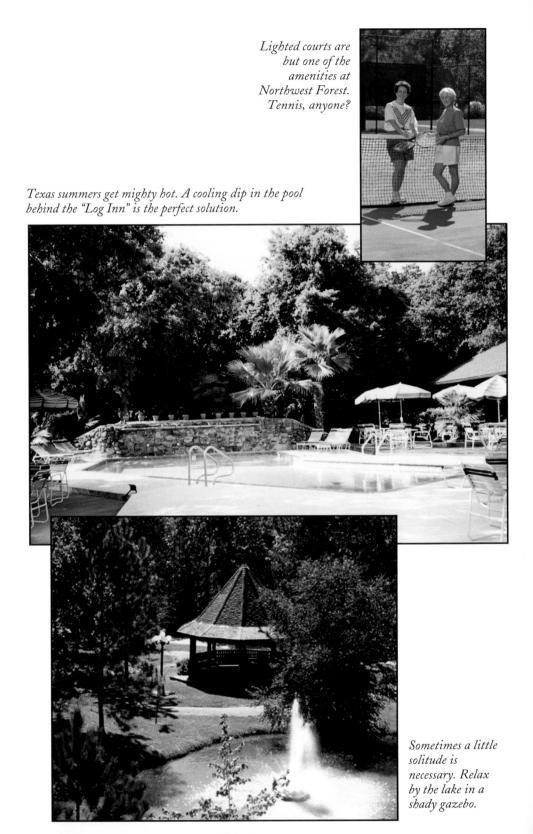

Lighted courts are but one of the amenities at Northwest Forest. Tennis, anyone?

Texas summers get mighty hot. A cooling dip in the pool behind the "Log Inn" is the perfect solution.

Sometimes a little solitude is necessary. Relax by the lake in a shady gazebo.

Lord, Don't Let Me Sneeze... or Cough... or Laugh!

*N*early ten million women face the challenges of incontinence. To put it plainly, they wet their pants, suddenly and usually without much warning, and often in a public setting.

Causes may include pregnancy, childbirth, stress, menopause or age. In most cases, strengthening the pelvic floor muscles can relieve this embarrassing condition without surgical intervention. And it can be done in the privacy of a woman's own home.

Sadly, it is estimated that only 1 in 12 ever seek help, according to Dr. Dante Marinelli, a urologist and author of "Good News for Millions With Incontinence."

There are essentially three types of incontinence: stress incontinence, urge incontinence and overflow incontinence, and sometimes a combination.

Stress Incontinence

This is the most common type and occurs when you leak urine upon coughing, laughing or exercising. Additional pressure on the abdomen and bladder from sports, exercising, lifting something heavy like groceries or a toddler, or sometimes just a cough or sneeze, may result in urine leakage.

One study indicated that one in three women experienced this type of incontinence during exercise, and 20% stopped exercising as a result. Because exercise is essential to general good health for everyone, incontinence can quickly become not only inconvenient and embarrassing, but also unhealthy.

Urge Incontinence

This is the inability to hold your urine long enough to get to the bathroom. Women with this type incontinence often go to the bathroom every two hours, or more often, just to prevent accidents. These frequent trips to the bathroom, especially for women who work outside the home or who travel, often generate unwanted jokes and comments, with resulting anxiety.

Hearing "gee, your bladder must only hold a teaspoon!" for the 500th time requires all the restraint a woman can muster to keep from clobbering the insensitive speaker. It also may cause a woman to avoid social events for fear of having an accident.

Overflow Incontinence

This is when you get up frequently during the night to go to the bathroom, or take a long time to urinate and have a weak, dribbling stream with no force. Even though you urinate in small amounts, you may not feel completely "empty." If this condition persists, it can interfere with healthy sleep patterns and will most certainly cause anxiety.

Mixed Incontinence

A combination of stress and urge incontinence frequently occurs together, especially in older women following menopause.

Cause of Incontinence

Because there are many causes of incontinence, a woman should not feel guilty for something she literally has little or no control over. As an example, childbirth or a chronic cough can lead to incontinence. There's not a whole lot a woman can do to prevent incontinence during the time these events are taking place.

Frequent constipation or excess weight both contribute to incontinence. While steps can be taken to address these factors, they can not be eliminated instantly. Often these conditions occur during pregnancy and continue for a time following childbirth.

Some medications for depression, high blood pressure, heart disease and insomnia have been shown to cause incontinence. Conditions such as Parkinson's, stroke or diabetes can also damage the nerves that control the bladder.

First Stop Is Your Doctor's Office

A physician can determine if there are underlying medical reasons for incontinence, such as overactive bladder muscles, a malfunction of the urinary sphincter or a urinary tract infection. So see your physician first to rule out these things. Your next stop should be your nearest Women's Health Boutique.

WHB professionals have been trained in incontinence management, and are available to discuss this condition privately and confidentially. The boutiques carry a variety of products, including a biofeedback device and vaginal cones, or weights, both used to help strengthen the pelvic floor muscles.

There's also a selection of feminine panties and liners, enabling a woman to buy these products confidentially and without embarrassment. Specialty skin care products to ease skin discomfort and address odor problems are available, too, along with information on how best to use them.

Find the freedom to resume an active lifestyle, without fear of embarrassment ever again. No woman suffering from incontinence should have to hide at home when a solution is as near as Women's Health Boutique.

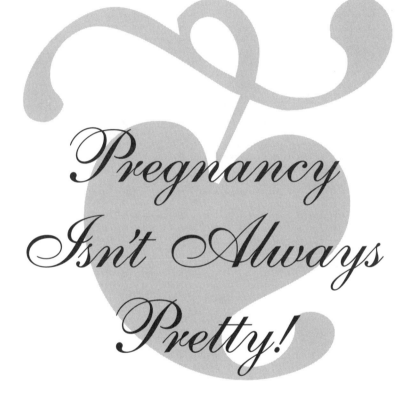

Pregnancy Isn't Always Pretty!

*W*ow! I'm pregnant! I'm going to have a baby!

There's no greater thrill in a woman's life than when she says those words…I'm going to have a baby. She thinks of tiny little dresses and delicate little booties. She carefully unpacks the hand-made blanket her grandmother made and starts thinking about what color the nursery should be. She feels beautiful and special.

Then her ankles swell, and her bra doesn't fit right, and her tummy starts to itch and her back hurts. That's when she realizes—pregnancy isn't always pretty.

But, she's still going to have a baby, so what can she do to make it through the nine months? After the initial visit to her obstetrician, where can she go to get all the "stuff" she needs to make her life easier?

Women's Health Boutique carries an extensive inventory of specialty products designed just for the mother-to-be. Whether a woman works outside the home or not—and over 75% of women do work into their third trimester—it is essential that she utilize any of the products that will make her feel more comfortable. This is especially important because she can't always rest for a few minutes or put her feet up.

Varicose veins can develop or worsen during pregnancy due to increased weight, blood volume and hormonal changes. Light pressure maternity compression hose will relieve leg fatigue and swollen ankles. For more severe varicose veins or persistent swelling, a woman's doctor may prescribe stronger compression hosiery or tights. The boutiques carry a full line of maternity hosiery, and consultants can help a woman learn how to put on the hosiery for maximum benefit.

Lower back pain is another common complaint during pregnancy. A properly fitted maternity belt, girdle or lumbo-sacral support, all available at WHB, relieve abdominal and pelvic pressure and help reduce the low back pain.

Along about the fourth or fifth month of pregnancy, the mother-to-be will want to have one of the certified fitters at WHB help her choose a properly fitted maternity bra. Maternity bras, unlike conventional lingerie, are designed to expand with breasts and rib cage during pregnancy. The bra should be comfortable at the tightest hook so that it will allow for expansion during the remainder of the pregnancy. A professional fitter will make sure the bra fits correctly.

Just choosing a larger size non-maternity bra will not give the necessary extra support during pregnancy, nor will a regular bra allow for growth as the pregnancy progresses. This is a case where trying to cut corners is not wise, and could cause fatigue and discomfort during a very special time in a woman's life.

Experts also agree that the same bra should not be worn for maternity and nursing. The bra worn during pregnancy may become worn or stretched and will fail to provide the support needed to be effective when worn later as a nursing bra.

And what about those dreaded stretch marks? Will this pregnancy mean the end of two piece bathing suits? Will a permanent road map be etched across the tummy? Not at all!

Pregnancy not only changes the body, but it creates new challenges for the skin. As the body expands, the skin stretches. Effective moisturizing is essential to keep the skin hydrated. A rich emollient recovery cream adds needed moisture to help prevent those once inevitable stretch marks. There's a wonderful massage oil, fortified with moisturizers, in WHB's specialty skin care products. This is an excellent product for overall body care, not only during pregnancy but beyond.

Not to be forgotten during this special time is the wonderful selection of lingerie, wigs and turbans. There's no reason to feel dowdy or unattractive, night or day. And on those "bad hair days," it's great to have an already styled wig to pop on, or a stylish wrap.

Thanks to Women's Health Boutique, pregnancy can be pretty.

Breast Feeding Isn't Always Fun

*N*early 70% of all new mothers today choose to breastfeed. And why not? Breast milk provides perfectly balanced nutrition for your baby and is ideally suited for a baby's immature digestive system.

Breastfeeding is beneficial to both mother and baby. Your baby receives important immune resistance to allergens and illness through breast milk. And, breastfeeding helps the uterus contract to the pre-pregnancy size more quickly.

The hormone prolactin, which stimulates relaxation, is produced during breastfeeding, and those quiet intimate moments several times a day, with just mother and baby, can have a life-long effect for both.

But what if breastfeeding isn't the beautiful experience you thought it would be? What if it hurts too much, or your baby seems to reject the breast? What if you don't have the slightest idea how to go about it, and you've decided you're the worst possible mother because it doesn't come "naturally" to you? Or, what if you're an expectant mother and want to learn all you can about this very important first step in mothering?

Women's Health Boutique is just the place for you. The Educational Library in each boutique offers a selection of books, videotapes and literature about successful breastfeeding. These resources may be checked out free of charge, allowing you to review these materials in the privacy of your home. People who genuinely care about you will answer any questions you may have.

Many busy mothers-on-the-go may want to use a breast pump for baby's nourishment while mother and baby are separated, or when traveling. Everything a new mother will need for breastfeeding is available at WHB. You can choose between several styles of breast pumps, for either purchase or short-term rental, storage bags and a carrying case/cooler.

Lactation consultants help guide mother and baby through the joys of breastfeeding, and can advise strategies that will work best for any situation. This is especially important with the current trend of sending new mothers home from the hospital within a couple of days after giving birth.

Nursing mothers need the support of a professionally fitted nursing bra. A certified fitter at the boutique will assist new or expectant mothers in finding just the right one. This is an important step in future good health and shouldn't be left to chance at a self-help lingerie counter.

WHB carries an excellent line of skin care products, and can even offer creams to help heal sore, chapped or cracked nipples. Nursing pads are available to help the nursing mother stay comfortable between feedings. For those mothers with retracted nipples, a trained consultant will help her select breast shells to make breastfeeding easier.

This is a special time for new mothers, and even for experienced mothers. Women's Health Boutique can help you and your baby make beautiful memories as you choose what's best for you.

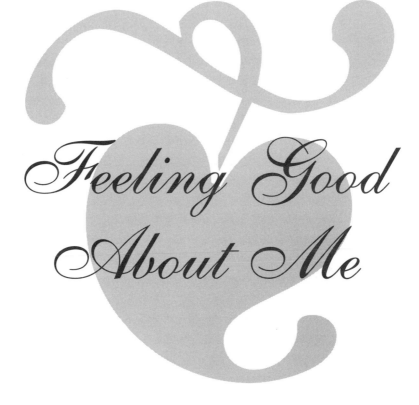

Feeling Good
About Me

*E*very woman should be able to face each day with eager-
ness, confident that she looks and feels her best. While
many women may never experience a catastrophic health
crisis, every woman will almost certainly have health and image
concerns that deserve to be addressed.

It's comforting to know that Women's Health Boutique is there
to help women handle those stressful situations.

The Right Bra

It has been estimated that 8 out of 10 women wear an incor-
rectly fitted bra. This is not only uncomfortable, but can cause
health problems. Back strain is a common result of wearing the
wrong bra. Constriction of a too-tight band or cup may also put
pressure on the lymph glands. Some medical professionals are
even beginning to suspect ill-fitting bras may contribute to the
formation of breast tumors.

The professional fitters at WHB will help each woman find
the proper size bra for comfort and health. Not every woman
should wear the same size bra she wore twenty—or even five—
years ago. She will be much more comfortable in a size that's right
for her as she is today.

Having a bra professionally fitted is of particular interest to
small-breasted or large-breasted women who may find it difficult
to find the correct bra in self-service department stores. Women's
Health Boutique carries a full inventory of bras from the smaller
sizes to 46J, or larger, and can help any woman find the right fit.
Fittings are done discreetly in the private fitting rooms at WHB.

Skin Care

Skin care is a necessity throughout a woman's life. With all the
attention being given to protecting our skin from environmental
attacks, it is important to have products readily available to take
care of this highly visible part of our body.

The excellent skin care line at WHB features products for every stage of a woman's life. General skin care products, including those with ultraviolet protection, help a woman maintain the health of her skin. During pregnancy there are special creams to smooth on the stretching skin to ease discomfort and minimize stretch marks. And for those confined to bed due to accident or infirmity, there are several products designed to relieve skin discomfort and to aid in personal cleansing.

Banish Bad Hair Days

Every woman has experienced a "bad hair day," a day when no amount of coaxing can make a hairstyle look right. A visit to a Women's Health Boutique can banish those days forever. Each WHB has a wonderful selection of wigs that look and feel like real hair and can be styled right there in the boutique by a trained cosmetologist. Just by popping on a wig, or choosing a stylish turban or wrap, a woman can greet the day feeling confident and attractive.

Having a wig or a wrap on standby is like having the right accessories for a favorite ensemble. It allows a woman to look and feel her best, regardless of the circumstances. Each boutique carries a complete inventory of wig care products, and a consultant will give tips on caring for the wig.

Plastic/Cosmetic Surgery Assistance

Using makeup and hair styling to achieve a desired look is important to a woman. But there are times when she may want to be a bit more aggressive in her approach to her image. With the advances in cosmetic surgery, this solution is being chosen more frequently. Women's Health Boutique professionals have the knowledge and the products to provide a significant part of the after-care following these procedures.

Post operative compression garments, offering refined and elegant styling, are designed to meet the ever changing field of plastic/reconstructive surgery. For either a minor procedure or an extensive one, the staff at Women's Health Boutique can provide the necessary garments recommended by the physician.

Intended to be put on in the operating room and worn for a period of days or weeks, these garments offer all-important support for delicate tissues following this type surgery. Some garments are designed with special zippers, allowing change without pulling and tugging that can cause damage to reconstructed areas. The fabric is a breathable power net, and comes in white, black or champagne, so a woman can still feel feminine during recovery.

There are several garments ideally suited for use after breast reduction, augmentation or reconstruction. These range from simple breast wraps to full torso garments when the surgery involves adjoining tissues. The type garment is chosen by the physician for optimum support, but the style helps a woman feel attractive during the healing process.

Facial compression wear is used for many purposes, including the popular facelifts and facial liposuction. Other facial surgeries, such as chin-jowl augmentation, or similar implants, require use of facial support garments. Facial compression garments are also used following accidental trauma, for TMJ surgery and therapy, after oral surgery, and even as an anti-snoring device.

Whether a woman needs a simple three-inch breast wrap, a chest-to-ankle garment, or some type of facial band, Women's Health Boutique can provide the appropriate compression wear.

Supports and Braces

If a support device is needed, Women's Health Boutique is the first place to go. There are many reasons a support device may be needed, and there are many products on the market. A doctor may prescribe a back brace, called an orthosis, if back strain has resulted from lifting or performing a strenuous task. An ankle brace aids in the healing of sprains and strains, or after a cast has been removed, and can also be worn to support weak ankles during vigorous activity, such as aerobics.

Posture supports encourage proper positioning of back and shoulders and help relieve discomfort. For those suffering from carpal tunnel syndrome, arthritis or wrist strain, specially designed wrist braces relieve stress on the affected muscles and tendons.

And of course, WHB carries a complete line of support hosiery, not just for expectant mothers, but for any woman with special needs. Today's compression hosiery is available in fashionable colors and styles, and there's even a special stocking aid to make donning them easier.

Today's woman wants and needs services and products that help her maintain a healthy outlook on life. No matter what the need, both she and her doctor can be assured of professional care at Women's Health Boutique.

Section

2

Now let us share with you the stories of some of the people who have been helped by Women's Health Boutique and the difference it made in their lives...

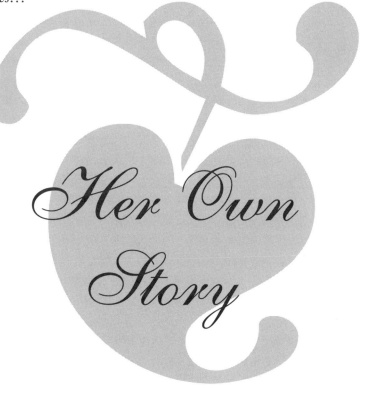

Her Own Story

*Names have been changed to protect the privacy of the individuals depicted.

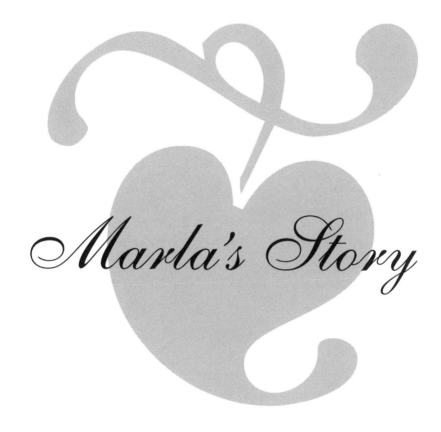

Marla's Story

*M*arla slipped into the Women's Health Boutique quietly. That's how she moved these days... quietly, so no one would notice her. Since "the surgery" as she had begun to call it, she hoped no one would notice her ever again. Why should they? She was mutilated, ugly. Why should they notice her? Why would they?

As Karen approached, Marla cringed, thinking of how to tell this woman, this whole woman, why she was here. This is a mistake, thought Marla. I shouldn't have come here. I should just go home and stay there. I don't know how to be *me* anymore.

But now Karen was right there, smiling, asking how she could help Marla. How indeed? Marla still remembered walking into that lingerie shop downtown to buy—she couldn't bring herself to say the word. It's just that after "the surgery," there was nothing —*there.* She felt lopsided, as if she would topple over any minute. Even when she took a deep breath, there was no movement, no life. Part of her was gone, and nothing, nothing she could buy in a store, would ever make that okay.

Marla stammered her way through an explanation, whispering that ugly, ugly word the doctors used. To her horror, she found herself telling Karen of the pain she felt walking into that shop with all the beautiful silky things that she could never wear again...ever. She told of making her way through the racks, brushing against the soft fabric, remembering how it felt to slip into something feminine and sexy and...revealing.

And then she burst into tears as she told of being taken into the shop manager's office at that other place and being asked to reveal—right there beside the desk!—the ugliness that remained so the clerk could see "what we're dealing with here." They sold the things and didn't even have a place—a private place—to undress!

She said all this to a stranger, her shoulders shaking with sobs for all she had lost. Not just the cancer. That she was glad to lose. But she mourned for that part of her that reminded her that she

I should just go home
and stay there.
I don't know how to be me
anymore.

was a woman. She mourned for the loss of her feminine self. She mourned that she could no longer wear a beautiful negligée that would cause Larry to catch his breath. She mourned for the Marla she used to be.

Karen put her arm around Marla and led her past beautiful lingerie, silky to the touch, cut perfectly to reveal and to conceal. She led her past swimsuits and blouses, wonderfully designed just for Marla. And then she led her to a cushioned loveseat and offered her a tissue.

As Marla sank back against the cushions, she felt hope slowly returning to her soul. She knew, she *knew,* that walking into Women's Health Boutique was a decision that would change the rest of her life.

Maybe, just maybe, she thought for the first time in many weeks, I'll feel like *me* again.

Granny Gets Bosoms

*E*velyn marched into the room, shoulders back, chin up and with just the slightest hint of a "look-at-me" smile. Perfectly coifed heads in various shades of gray, white and blue (and one implausible brunette) turned to watch their friend make her way to their usual table. Madge, Joyce and Fern sat waiting, mouths slightly agape, struck dumb in mid-conversation by the unusual demeanor of their usually shy luncheon companion and friend.

As she slipped into her chair, all three women leaned forward at once, just as they had 65 years ago when they whispered secrets under the wide front porch. You did it, hissed Fern, you really did it!

Yes I did, declared Evelyn. You *bet* I did! Whadda you think? Does it look funny? Can you tell? *WHAT DO YOU THINK?* The words tumbled out, tripping over one another as she sought approval from her life-long friends.

The three women sat there in the tea room where, for more years than memory could record, they had gathered for their monthly women's club luncheon. It was here they had exchanged stories of their children's school activities. They had shared their uncertainty about how to deal with teenagers. As the years passed, they passed around photos of their children and spouses and finally, grandchildren. It was in this room they had discussed their husbands, now gone.

It was also in this room 35 years ago they listened as Evelyn told them, voice quivering, that the doctor said she had cancer and he would have to remove her breasts—both of them. It was to this room that Evelyn came for her first real "outing" after the surgery. They had very carefully avoided looking below her chin that day, or any day after that, to the looseness, the emptiness, of her dress front.

But this day they looked. Very delicately, of course. Ladies nearing their eighth decade don't gawk at other people. But they looked, eyes widening as they recognized shape on Evelyn's chest.

*As Evelyn had dressed
that morning for her "debut,"
she felt like a girl again.
That's it, she thought,
I feel like a girl again!*

They saw roundness where it had been flat. As they looked from Evelyn's chest to one another, the same message flashed silently among them—Evelyn has **bosoms!**

As Evelyn had dressed that morning for her "debut," she felt like a girl again. That's it, she thought, I feel like a girl again! She was giddy as she chose just the right dress for the occasion. No more rolled up socks for her, no sir! These things feel *real,* she thought, trying to remember weight, and movement, on her chest. As she slipped her dress over her head and smoothed it down, she couldn't help cupping her hands over the roundness. Oh my, she thought, as her breath caught.

Then she jerked her hands away, suddenly feeling guilty, for what, she didn't know. She was grateful to be alive. That's what the doctor had told her she should feel on that awful day back in 1961. She had asked him what she was supposed to do now.

How was she supposed to find clothes to fit? What could she say to her husband? Would he even want to be married to her anymore?

She *was* grateful to be alive. Certainly she was grateful to be alive. But how she had missed wearing clothes that fit just so. How she had missed those parts of her that were gone. For a long time, she mourned for those lost parts. No, those parts didn't make her a woman. And not having them didn't make her less of a woman. But she missed them just the same.

And now, thanks to her precious granddaughter, she had those missing parts back again. She had—okay, Evelyn, say it because you're thinking it—she had bosoms again! And it felt *good.*

She had shared the beginning of this story with her three best friends, but they had not been with her when Denise took her downtown to the Women's Health Boutique for her first fitting. Denise understood her as none of her children or other grandchildren did, and somehow they had gotten into a conversation about her surgery so many years ago.

❦

---

*...having breasts or
not having breasts
does not make me a woman.
I'm still very much a
woman...a little flat maybe,
but at least I can sleep
on my stomach with
no problems!*

Denise asked her why, Granny, why didn't you have something done? Why didn't you ever get implants or falsies or **something?** Evelyn had explained to her that, back in the early '60's, death was usually the result of cancer like she had. There was little if any thought of whether clothes would fit or how it hurt emotionally to lose something that most people associate with being feminine.

She went on to explain that she had looked at "falsies," but they weren't any better than rolled up socks, which she already had at home. She told Denise that her husband David, Denise's grandfather, had never acted any differently toward her. He had remained gentle and loving and flattering, so most of the time she forgot the socks and just wore a soft cotton chemise under her dress. As for implants, there was never a thought about having that done. My dear, she chided Denise, in my day those were only done on—she lowered her voice to a whisper—actresses and such!

Besides, she said as she and Denise sat on the sun porch, having breasts or not having breasts does not make me a woman. I'm still very much a woman…a little flat, maybe, but at least I can sleep on my stomach with no problems! Denise laughed with her grandmother, but she couldn't quite let go of the notion that her wonderful grandmother deserved something, well, wonderful.

Denise worked for Women's Health Boutique, and talked to women and their caregivers every day about this sort of thing. The day after the chat with her grandmother, as Denise was preparing to visit with a patient care specialist at the local women's clinic, it came to her. I'll give Granny a new chest for Christmas! I'll get her a chest she'll love.

Two days later, Evelyn found herself in the fitting room at the local boutique. This lovely young woman with soft hands and caring eyes was fitting her for…what did they call them?…breast prostheses. Guess we don't call them falsies anymore, Evelyn laughed to herself.

That day was a blur, but the young woman very carefully helped her select the right undergarments from a fine selection. She escorted her to a fitting room, and with the utmost dignity, helped her into her new self.

Then this sweet lady hugged her! They were no longer strangers. They had shared a very special and irreplaceable moment of life. The hug was a most appropriate way to commemorate the occasion. Evelyn walked out of Women's Health Boutique with her shoulders back and her chin up and hasn't changed her posture since.

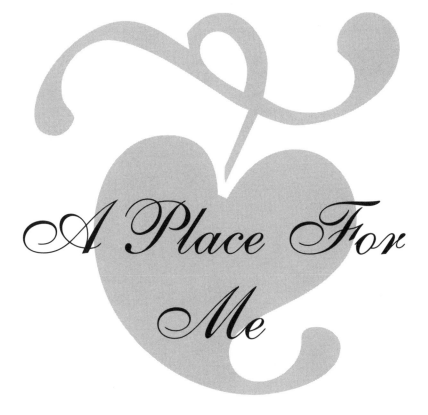

A Place For Me

*S*usan stood on the sidewalk for a few minutes looking through the windows of the Women's Health
Boutique. Finally, she took a deep breath and slowly
pulled the door open.

As she looked around the beautifully appointed room, her
eyes widened. She scanned the room, noticing the tasteful
displays, the lovely wigs and wraps against one wall, the swimsuits to her right. Her face, tense and drawn when she entered,
gradually relaxed. Judy had just approached her when Susan
broke into tears.

Judy instinctively put her arms around the sobbing woman's
shoulder and pulled her over to a comfortable chair. There, there,
she said, trying to comfort her. Everything's going to be okay.

Smiling through her tears, Susan grabbed Judy's hand and said
oh, I know it'll be okay *now*. I've found you! I've found you!

Introducing herself, Susan went on to explain. She had recently
had a mastectomy, and was only in the hospital a couple of days.
The whole sequence of events had happened so quickly that she
hardly had time to absorb the news that she had cancer. She
certainly had no time to plan for what she would do later.

Of course she had asked her doctor, but he could only suggest
vaguely that she find a "place" to buy breast forms and special
undergarments after her incision healed. He had given her no clue
as to where she could find this "place." So she had left the hospital with no idea what to do next.

Then a friend told her about Women's Health Boutique. As
she dried her tears, Susan exclaimed to Judy, I'm so glad I found
you! I just knew there had to be a place for me somewhere! This
is the place for me!

The first thing Judy did for Susan was take her to the
Educational Library area. Susan viewed a couple of short
videos to help her understand what had just happened to her
and what was ahead of her. Most doctors have literature available, but as Susan explained to Judy, sometimes it's hard to

understand some of the terminology, and the doctor is always so busy. The video selection at each boutique answers the questions a woman is likely to ask in clear, simple language.

Judy introduced Susan to the fine skin care products and described how they are used as the incision heals. Then she showed her the soft garment used while the skin is tender. The fiber-filled pockets offer shape but have no elastic bands or metal hooks to irritate sensitive skin.

They discussed the various breast prostheses on the market and how to choose the right one. Susan's eyes had continued to stray to the swimsuit display, so Judy showed her how the breast forms are worn in the hot tub, pool or even the ocean.

Two hours later, a smiling Susan floated out the door. She promised Judy she would be back to be fitted for her prosthesis and to pick out a swimsuit for her vacation in Acapulco.

Her parting words were I'm *so* glad I found you!

Yesterday I Couldn't Even Spell Mammography

*I may lose a breast,
but I don't have to die and
I don't have to give up
being pretty!*

*O*ctober—Breast Cancer Awareness Month. Every time Dorothy left home she saw a mobile mammography unit parked in a shopping center parking lot. Magazines carried articles about famous people who had "beaten" cancer. Newspapers covered the subject even more than usual. Billboards urging women to get mammograms seemed to be everywhere.

Dorothy had read the statistics, of course…44,000 women die every year from breast cancer. She knew that many women put off going for their first mammogram. She knew because she was one of them. Friends told horror stories about how much it hurt. Then she would read that it doesn't really hurt, it's just uncomfortable for a couple of minutes. Still, she put it off, and her doctor, not to mention some of her friends, were getting very impatient with her.

She opened her mailbox one September morning and found a brochure from a place called Women's Health Boutique. It was a pretty little advertisement, so she started reading it and discovered it was all about early detection of breast cancer through mammograms and self-exams. Included were guidelines for how to do a self-exam and what to look for, and a coupon offering a mammogram at one of the mobile units for only $55.

That evening while in the shower, Dorothy followed the instructions, and as her fingers slid tentatively across her wet skin, suddenly she felt…what? Oh, no! Not a lump! Yes, even as her heart pounded, Dorothy forced her fingers back to that spot. Sure enough, there was something…something alien…under the skin.

That night, Dorothy slept fitfully. At nine o'clock the next morning, fingers shaking, Dorothy dialed the number shown on the brochure for the mobile mammogram unit. A very kind woman answered. She explained the procedure, reassuring Dorothy that it would only be uncomfortable at best. Her steady voice calmed Dorothy. Maybe I'm just imagining this, Dorothy told herself. Maybe I didn't really feel anything at all!

Then the lady asked Dorothy about any lumps. Dorothy hesitated, then told her what she thought she had found. Still speaking calmly, the woman told Dorothy she should immediately make an appointment with her doctor, that the mammogram provided in the mobile unit was designed as a screening tool only, not for diagnosis.

She went on to assure Dorothy that she had found the lump early, and early detection is the key to long range successful treatment. As the conversation ended, she made Dorothy promise she would phone her own doctor.

Now, one week later, Dorothy entered the Women's Health Boutique, practically in shock. I'm having breast surgery in three days and I want to see everything you have. I want to know about breast prostheses, your wigs, even your nighties. I need to know I can be myself again, even if I do lose my breast!

As the consultant talked to Dorothy about the many different prostheses available, and showed her the beautifully designed lingerie, the whole story tumbled out.

You have saved my life. I wouldn't have found that lump in time without your brochure. And I wouldn't have known about all the wonderful things you have here. I feel very, very lucky, thanks to Women's Health Boutique. I may lose a breast, but I don't have to die, and I don't have to give up being pretty.

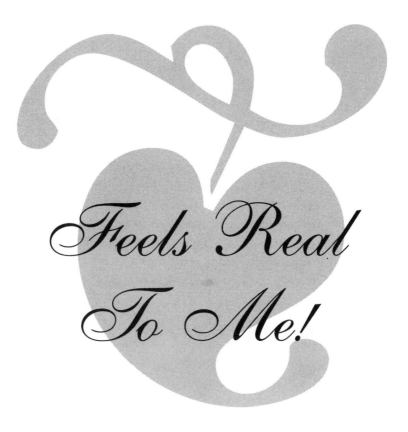

She stood in front of the mirror, marveling at the way her favorite dress now fit in front. Shyly, she stepped in front of her husband, almost whispering as she asked, well, what do you think?

*I*t isn't unusual for a husband and wife to come to Women's Health Boutique together, especially for the first visit. So when Richard and Betty walked in, Betty clutching Richard's hand until her knuckles turned white, Judy immediately set about making them feel at ease.

The story was familiar. Breast cancer. Mastectomy. Now Betty was so depressed about how she looked, especially to Richard, that it was almost painful to listen to her.

It was obvious how much the two cared for each other. It was also obvious that Betty thought Richard couldn't possibly feel the same toward her as he had before the surgery.

Judy introduced Betty to the certified mastectomy fitter and they retired to the fitting room. Richard sat in the waiting room area, but his eyes roamed the room, taking in all the beautiful lingerie, the stylish swimsuits, the wigs, and the various head wraps. He could have been sitting in almost any upscale shop waiting for his wife to show off her newest selection.

After a while, Betty came out of the fitting room. She stood a little taller and her eyes didn't seem so dark and pained. She paused in front of the mirror, marveling at the way her favorite dress now fit in front. Shyly, she stepped in front of her husband, almost whispering as she asked, well, what do you think?

Richard looked at his wife, adoration shining from his eyes. Slowly he got up and approached Betty. She caught her breath, not sure what would happen next.

He walked up to her, stopping just as his chest touched her arm. Then he reached out, and in a practiced move, pinched her new "breast!" With a wink and kiss on her cheek, Richard made her world start spinning again with a hearty *feels real to me!*

As Richard and Betty left, they were still holding hands, but this time as lovers, not survivors of some unbeatable battle. The staff cheered them, especially Richard, until the door closed behind them.

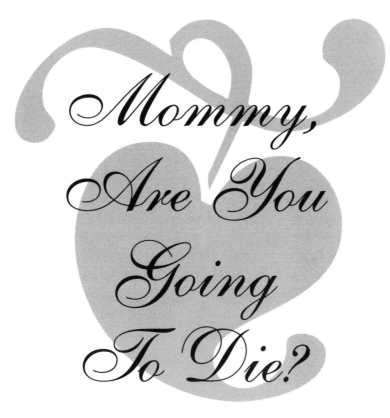

Mommy, Are You Going To Die?

*I*t was 2 o'clock in the afternoon when Linda came in the Women's Health Boutique, 8-year-old son Jason in tow. He was scowling and clearly not happy.

Linda, a scarf wrapped tastefully around her obviously bald head, installed Jason in the waiting area and told him to sit quietly while she looked at wigs.

Jason, however, had other ideas and proceeded to act on them. First he bounced on each of the chairs, pushing one against the wall with a thud. Then he took all of the brochures out of the rack, mixed them and returned them upside down.

Spying the clothes hanging on circular racks, Jason decided it would be great fun to play car wash, running under them with all the appropriate sound effects. Jason was, to put it mildly, a live wire.

Exasperated, Linda abandoned the fitting chair and grabbed Jason as he rushed by her. Jason! Whatever is the matter with you? Why can't you just sit over there as Mommy asked and be still?

Jason, his mother's hand firmly gripping his shoulder, looked up at his mother's face. Mommy, are you going to die? he asked loudly, his question echoing through the room.

Linda took his hand and led him back to the waiting area, pulling him up close. No, Jason, I'm not going to die. I just need to have some hair while I'm getting better.

But Mommy! One of my friends' mother got sick with that cancer stuff like you have and she died. Are you going to die too?

Oh, Jason, Linda sighed as she hugged her son tightly. Even if something did happen to me, you'll always have me with you in your heart.

Jason leaned against his mother, drawing strength from her calm words. Linda carefully disengaged from her son and asked him if he would now sit for a few minutes more while she looked at "hair." Jason nodded, his scowl replaced with almost a serene look. He sat quietly, taking in every person and every activity in the room while Linda returned to the wig counter.

Linda didn't find the "hair" she wanted that day, but she did buy a beautiful wrap to replace her scarf.

She collected the now calm Jason, and mother and son left the boutique, their smiling faces radiating their new stronger bond.

Section

3

PRODUCTS

Mastectomy
Breast forms ❧ Bras ❧ Custom fitting

Wigs
Hand tied ❧ Synthetic hair ❧ Special orders

Turbans
Comfortable ❧ Elegant ❧ Colorful ❧ Washable

Swimwear
One/two piece ❧ Accessories ❧ Plus Sizes

Compression
Comfortable ❧ Custom Fitting ❧ Durable

Advanced Skin Care
Sun protection ❧ Sensitivity free ❧ No preservatives

Incontinence
Panties ❧ Disposable undergarments & pads

Maternity
Bras/lingerie ❧ Support garments ❧ Breast pumps

MASTECTOMY
P R O D U C T S

After breast surgery, it's
important to find a place
that helps you feel like
yourself again. At
Women's Health Boutique,
you'll find a wide array of
breast forms – from
traditional to new and
innovative – that fulfill your
individual requirements
and unique needs.

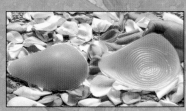

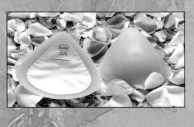

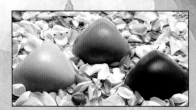

Complete selection
- Silicone
- Light and cool
- Attachable
- Custom

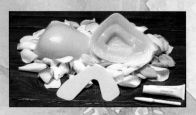

From leading manufacturers
- Amoena®
- Active®
- Camp
- Nearly Me®
- Airway®
- Jodee®

MASTECTOMY
PRODUCTS

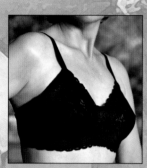

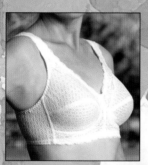

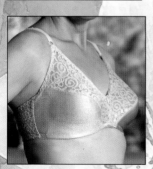

For the longest time, women thought mastectomy bras were unattractive. Not any more!

Women's Health Boutique has lovely bras in all sizes and colors. Come in for a custom fitting, because being comfortable is as important as looking good.

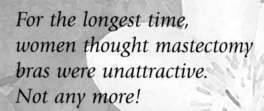

- *Front closure*
- *Posture support*
- *Non-wire underwire*
- *Long-line*
- *Built-in pockets*
- *Camisole*

WIGS & TURBANS

Whether you are undergoing chemotherapy or need a solution for thinning hair, we can help you regain confidence and create the look you desire.

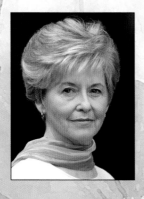

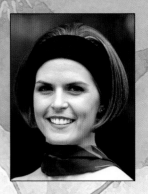

- Hand tied
- Natural part
- Synthetic
- Human hair
- Face framers
- Bangs
- Special orders

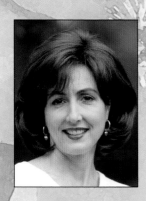

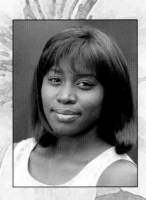

WIGS & TURBANS

We care about how you look. Whether you're going
out or staying home, we will teach you to easily
coordinate headwear with the rest of your wardrobe.
Check out our hats, scarves and sleep caps too!

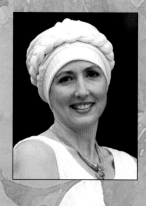

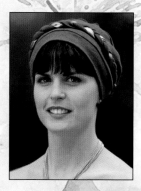

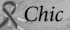

Chic

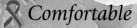

Comfortable

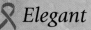

Elegant

Flattering

Colorful

Washable

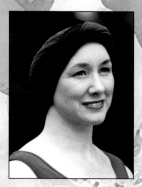

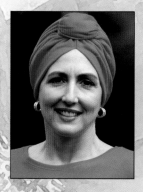

MASTECTOMY
SWIMWEAR

*Shopping for a swimsuit can be a challenge.
Women's Health Boutique makes this difficult
and sometimes frustrating task a little easier, all
in a private and comfortable atmosphere.*

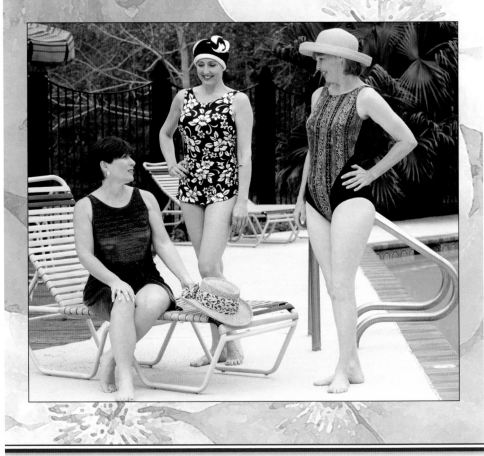

MASTECTOMY SWIMWEAR

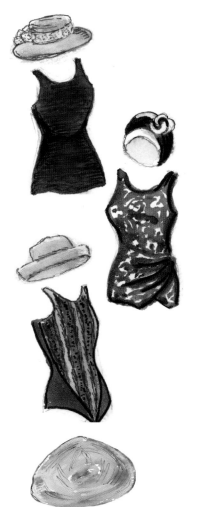

Every swimsuit has pockets that hold breast forms in place. Perfect for lounging by the pool, water aerobics or relaxing in the spa.

- ✺ *One-piece & Two-piece*
- ✺ *Sarong/Skirt*
- ✺ *High cut*
- ✺ *Plus sizes*

Add a foam or silicone swim form that's made to withstand chlorine and saltwater.

COMPRESSION

Swelling in your arms and legs can be painful and, if left untreated, can cause serious problems. Our therapeutic compression systems help alleviate the discomfort and effects of leg fatigue, varicose veins and post-surgery lymphedema.

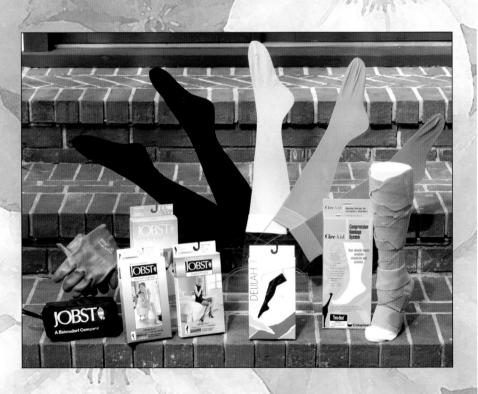

COMPRESSION

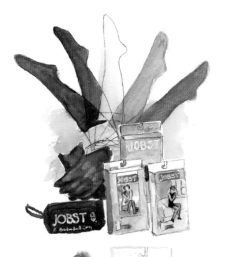

We have the highest quality compression garments from the most-recognized names in the industry, including Jobst®, Juzo®, Sigvaris® and Circaid®.

- 💥 Comfortable
- 💥 Custom fitting available
- 💥 Durable
- 💥 Ultra sheer hosiery
- 💥 Knee-high, Thigh-high & Waist-high
- 💥 Maternity

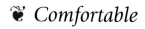

ADVANCED
SKIN CARE

Protecting skin is essential for every woman. Our advanced skin care products restore dry, sensitive skin resulting from cancer treatment or diabetes. Irritation from incontinence can be relieved for hours, and our moisturizers are great for maintaining completely healthy skin.

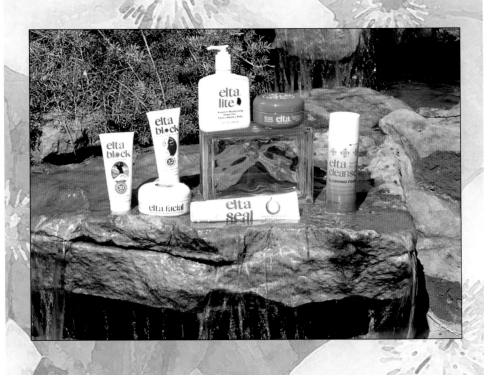

ADVANCED
S K I N   C A R E

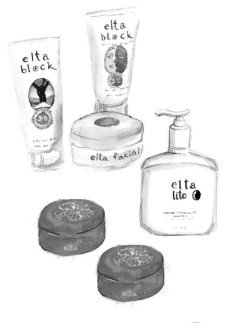

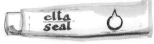

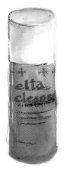

Water evaporates off the skin unless it is sealed in, while soap strips natural oils that maintain moisture. We can help your skin stay soft and moist.

* *Fragrance free*
* *Melts on contact*
* *Fast acting*
* *Broad spectrum sun protection*
* *Long lasting*
* *Sensitivity free*
* *No preservatives*

INCONTINENCE

Women's Health Boutique has products for your delicate personal and hygiene needs, including stress incontinence and bladder control. Our thoughtful staff is always sensitive to your privacy.

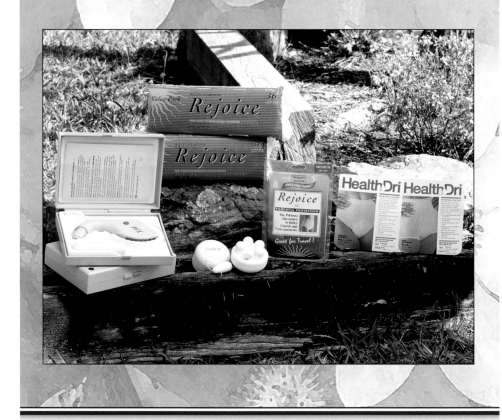

INCONTINENCE

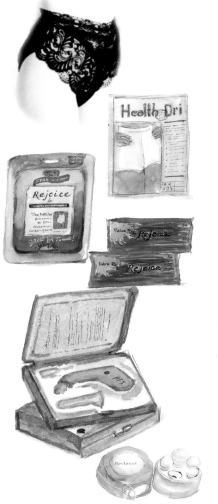

There are solutions for managing the challenge of incontinence.

- ❧ *Washable panties*
- ❧ *Disposable undergarments*
- ❧ *Disposable pads*
- ❧ *Pelvic muscle exercisers*
- ❧ *Vaginal weights*
- ❧ *Advanced skin care products*

MATERNITY

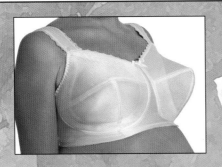

In your second trimester, we will professionally fit you for pre-natal bras that provide extra support for your growing figure.

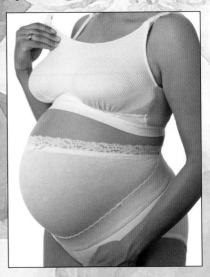

We can help alleviate your abdominal and lower back pains with maternity support panties and support belts that provide feminine comfort.

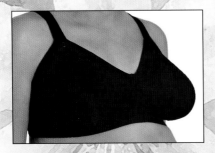

As delivery nears and excitement grows, let us professionally fit you for nursing bras.

MATERNITY

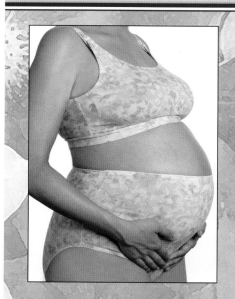

Our elegant lingerie comes in many styles to help maintain your expression of beauty.

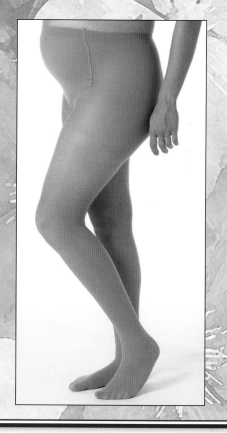

With your doctor's guidance, we will accurately measure you for compression hosiery designed to prevent varicose veins and swelling.

MATERNITY

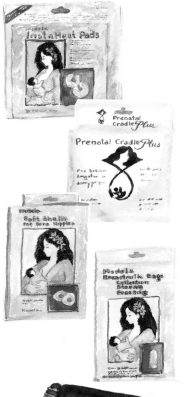

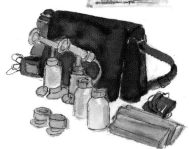

Whether you're a first-time mom or an experienced mom, come see our impressive collection.

- ❦ *Maternity bras to size JJ*
- ❦ *Educational Library*
- ❦ *Trusted names like Medela®, White River, Pre-Natal Cradle®, Ameda/Egnell and more*
- ❦ *Electric breast pump rental or purchase*
- ❦ *Battery operated pumps*
- ❦ *Maternity compression hosiery*

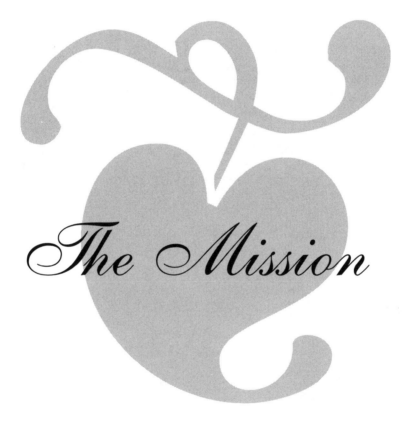

The Mission

*W*omen's Health Boutique has been called the 'Victoria's Secret' of healthcare, but that doesn't begin to describe what this business really is.

Focusing exclusively on women's health, WHB is really a healthcare provider in a unique retail setting.

The mission is simple: To meet the special healthcare needs of women, and to make a positive difference in the way women look and feel about themselves.

This is accomplished by providing a warm, feminine and comforting boutique environment with highly trained, compassionate staff who genuinely care about meeting each woman's special needs.

A woman may be experiencing a disease such as breast cancer, along with the needs associated with that. She may have skin care problems, osteoporosis or incontinence. She may be dealing with lymphedema, hair loss from radiation, chemotherapy, medication or disease. Perhaps she has fatigued legs or swollen ankles, is pregnant, or is dealing with a multitude of other conditions. WHB is there to help her handle these difficult situations.

Each boutique carries a variety of products designed to meet a woman's special needs. For post-breast surgery, there are camisoles, radiation garments, breast forms, bras and lingerie, wigs and turbans, swimwear and swim forms, partial forms and enhancers, compression garments and more.

There are products for women with pregnancy, postnatal and breastfeeding needs—prenatal bras, maternity girdles, back supports, nursing bras and breast pumps.

Women's personal care needs are met with bladder control and incontinence management products. There are specialty bras and skin care products, especially those used after surgery, even such elective surgeries as liposuction. For the woman who has difficulty finding a properly fitted bra in a department store, skilled bra fitters are on staff to help her.

For physicians and other healthcare professionals, Women's Health Boutique can complete their circle of care by offering special health-related products in a beautiful boutique designed for privacy and comfort.

These product choices can and do enhance a woman's lifestyle, enabling her to resume her life and activities without suffering embarrassment and discomfort.

WHB provides excellence in women's health products and services through preferred provider relationships in managed care organizations. The system is set up to handle third-party payments from various managed care plans, private insurance and Medicare.

Prostheses, mastectomy bras, compression hosiery, wigs, breast pumps and other products are often reimbursable. WHB staff members help clients determine which items are covered and will assist in processing insurance claims.

Today's woman wants and needs information about her particular health concerns. Founder Vicki D. Jones tells women, "Knowledge is the power that enables you to take charge of your healing process, rather than letting someone else tell you what to do."

For that reason, each boutique has an Educational Library filled with books, videos and audio tapes that women can check out and take home. The boutiques also offer facilities for support groups, participate in health fairs and are involved in other community education projects.

Vicki is often asked why she and her sister, Seleta, started this particular business.

"We started it because no woman should ever settle for second best when it comes to health and dignity."

"We started it for all the survivors of breast cancer who need one place to go for everything they should have to make them feel pretty again, a place where they're treated with respect and dignity."

"We deal with products for incontinence management because I've been plagued with this condition for years. Yes, it strikes younger women, too! I've been embarrassed many times over because I didn't know it could be managed without surgery. I sure didn't want to just sit home and hide, and I knew other women didn't want to either!"

"When women come into one of the boutiques for the first time," says Vicki, "they are overwhelmed by the high level of service and the caring attitude that permeates every aspect of the operation."

"In many cases, women have gone without a product that could help them because they didn't know it existed. Sometimes they've even been told they'll just have to live with it."

"That makes me angry, because no woman should have to 'live with' a condition that is manageable. When these women find us, they are surprised and delighted with the atmosphere and the vast range of products and services."

"Our ongoing commitment to women's health education and research, our continued involvement on state and national levels, and our commitment to excellence in franchising will keep WHB on the cutting edge of women's health."

"There are women everywhere who deserve more, and Women's Health Boutique is going to provide what they need."

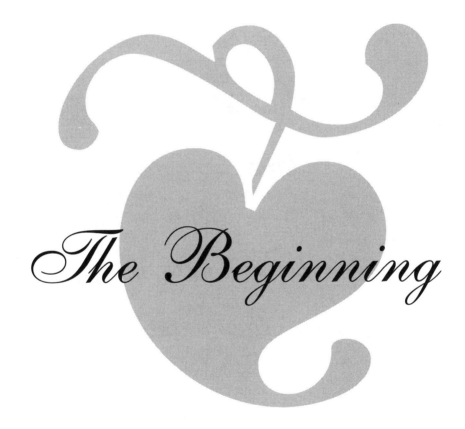

The Beginning

*"Every night
I go home feeling like
I have done something special
for another woman."*

*T*hese words by Vicki Dortch Jones, founder of Women's Health Boutique Franchise Systems, Inc. capture the spirit of the franchise devoted exclusively to women's health.

WHB was conceived in tragedy…the illness and death of one woman. But what a difference that one woman made!

Billie Dortch was a woman with a passion for business in an era when most women stayed home, raised mannerly children, baked cookies and sat quietly beside their husbands at business dinners.

Then in 1986, she was told she had cancer, caused by a diagnostic drug she was given thirty years before that was known even then to be toxic. The cancer would prove to be fatal. Even though they may never know her name, women across the country can be grateful to Billie Dortch, because her needless death sparked the creation of Women's Health Boutique.

With her death, she passed on her legacy of service, and her medical equipment business, to her daughters Vicki Jones and Seleta Lovell. Both young women were involved in their own families and careers, but the opportunity to continue their mother's business was one they couldn't refuse. The sisters joined forces and began learning, day by day, on-the-job, the home medical equipment trade.

Each woman gravitated to a different area of service to their customers. Having worked closely with her mother, Seleta now assumed management of the daily operations, while Vicki handled customer sales, marketing and advertising. The sisters prided themselves on customer service that was second to none.

Fed by the frustration they experienced trying to find products and services for their mother during her illness, they began exploring ways to do something for other women so they wouldn't have to do without the things their mother had so desperately needed.

They dedicated a corner of the showroom for a creatively designed mastectomy area, sort of a corner boutique. From that small beginning sprang Women's Health Boutique, one of the more unique concepts in women's healthcare today.

One day Marty Thacker came through the door, and an idea was born. Thirty-nine years old, Marty had chronic lymphedema in her arm following a radical mastectomy several years earlier. Vicki hired her as a women's consultant, on a part-time basis because of her health.

At that time, women visiting the boutique area had to make their way past wheelchairs and hospital beds, a very cold and clinical path. Vicki expressed her wish to Marty that the atmosphere be more like the elegant lingerie shop in town that also sold breast forms.

Marty had been in that other shop, shortly after her mastectomy. She had walked past all the beautiful and revealing lingerie she could no longer wear, to the back of the shop.

She had relayed her request to the sales clerk and was shown the small selection of breast forms. When she asked about being fitted, the clerk seemed puzzled for a moment, and finally invited Marty into the cluttered office next to the stockroom.

It was at that point that Marty realized she was expected to disrobe right there in the office, exposing her surgical scars amidst the paper clips to a woman who obviously had no training in fitting mastectomy patients, and who didn't even notice her pain. Marty fled the shop.

Years later, as she related that awful experience, tears ran down her cheeks, the pain still fresh and raw.

That day was a turning point. As Vicki helped Marty dry her tears, she promised her, "One day I'll have a store just as beautiful as that lingerie shop, but it will be totally devoted to meeting your needs and every woman like you."

Less than six months later, in February 1991, the first Women's

Health Boutique opened in the space adjoining the medical equipment store. Sadly, Marty didn't live to see what she had inspired.

As word spread of this wonderful place, women would travel for hours to shop there because their needs were so obviously not being met elsewhere.

Vicki and Seleta discovered that many inadequacies existed in the various areas of women's health, especially for women with pregnancy, childbirth and breastfeeding needs, and for women experiencing urinary incontinence. Products designed to meet those challenges were added to the inventory.

They listened to their customers. They learned to ask women what they wanted, when they wanted it, and how they wanted it. They learned that women hungered for information, for education, for answers. Always in their thoughts was their proud, independent mother, slowly stripped of her dignity because no one knew where to turn for help.

As word spread about this unique service to women, people would fly in from all over the country to look at the successful boutique the two sisters operated in Longview, Texas, wanting the same thing in their own town.

It was then that the women realized it was time to take the next step in growing the business, and so began studying expansion strategies.

Franchising, they quickly came to understand, offered the perfect solution for getting out the company's mission, which, simply stated, is to restore dignity to women everywhere who need these services, and help them return to healthy, productive lives.

They found themselves at the helm of a business phenomenon, and with the enthusiasm those near them had come to expect, they steered it straight into the pages of business history.

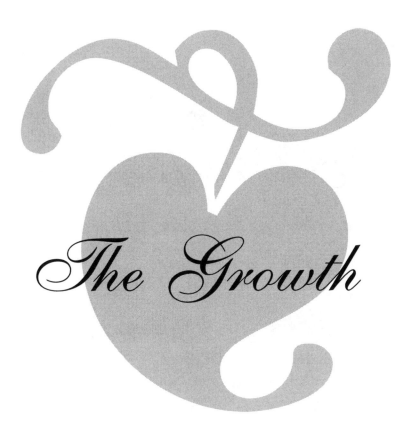

The Growth

"Growth that is too good can be just as dangerous as no growth at all."

Cassity Jones, successful entrepreneur and
Vicki D. Jones' father-in-law

*W*omen's Health Boutique started growing by leaps and bounds. Not only was the original boutique in East Texas booming, national publicity was drawing more and more people there clamoring for a chance at this unique franchising opportunity.

No longer was this a small-town operation. There was a corporate staff. Marketing had to be done, a training curriculum devised, support provided.

The workload was enormous, and the growing pains of this new business were being felt very deeply.

It had seemed so simple. This was a successful business; others wanted to do the same thing, so why not franchise? Now it was beginning to seem as though this franchise cart had gotten ahead of the knowledge horse.

Vicki had affiliated with the leading franchise groups in the country. As she attended meetings, she made it a point to seek out the leaders in the field to ask their advice and counsel.

"I always tried to do exactly what my mentor suggested. If I didn't plan on listening and doing what they said, I wouldn't ask." She went on to admit, "Unfortunately, when I was given sound advice, unsolicited, I seldom listened."

Perhaps that's why she didn't heed her father-in-law's advice the first time he said it. Cassity Jones is a successful businessman himself, patriarch of a chain of hardware, home improvement and lumber stores dotting the East Texas landscape.

His business philosophy—almost his motto—is that "growth that is too good can be just as dangerous as no growth at all." In other words, a business can grow too fast to handle well, and that's just as dangerous as not growing at all.

Vicki was beginning to realize the wisdom of his words. "I thought about quitting. My children needed me, my husband needed me. But hundreds of thousands of women needed me, too. Women who had nowhere to turn needed me to help them face…and conquer…the health challenges thrown at them."

That's when she met franchising giants Bud Hadfield and Steve Hammerstein. Bud is a legend in franchising, having founded Kwik Kopy Printing in the 1960's. He heads the International Center for Entrepreneurial Development—ICED for short—the parent company for an alliance of franchises spread throughout 15 countries.

Steve Hammerstein, president and CEO of ICED, was, at the time Vicki met him, chairman of the International Franchise Association, the world's oldest and largest franchising trade group.

"Their mentoring gave me renewed strength and faith," says Vicki. "It all started when I read Bud's book, *Wealth Within Reach.* I wanted to throw in the towel, but Bud's honesty, his experience, his perseverance, and his success, inspired me beyond degree."

"The day I finished his book, I wrote Bud Hadfield and told him *I will never, never, never, never give up!*"

Bud and Steve mentored Vicki for 19 months, guiding her through the treacherous waters of franchising and business ownership. But when Women's Health Boutique began to spread nationwide, Vicki decided it was time to join forces with someone who could communicate the mission on a larger scale.

She knew that, for continued growth and expansion, she needed the financial strength, the management expertise, and the vast experience in franchising of someone else.

The "someone" was obvious. Bud, Steve and the ICED organization recognized the tremendous opportunity offered by this new and exciting concept in the rapidly changing healthcare industry.

In 1996, ICED acquired WHB, consolidating it into a family of franchises with annual revenues of just under $18 million and an infrastructure of support and marketing exceeded by no one.

Women's Health Boutique, the only system focusing exclusively on women's health issues, was now positioned to achieve its full potential as an international player and carry its mission to women around the world.

Section

4

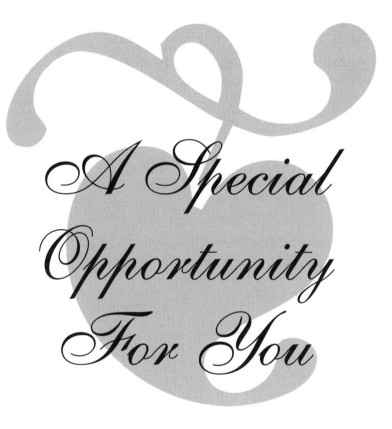

*A Special
Opportunity
For You*

*W*omen's Health Boutique is one of the most unique franchising opportunities available today, and is in a virtually untapped market. Plus, it has phenomenal growth potential.

Every woman is a potential customer of the boutiques, regardless of her age or station in life. Every woman will face some sort of health challenge in her lifetime. Every woman knows another woman who is concerned about some aspect of her health right now.

These women deserve to have a boutique in their community, or at least nearby, so their concerns can be addressed. They deserve to live a full life, unfettered by health issues that keep them from doing so.

Perhaps you have been thinking about a different direction for your life, one that allows you more opportunities for personal service. Or, maybe you have been looking for a business for yourself, a business where you're in charge and where you have more freedom to make decisions.

ICED welcomes inquiries into franchise opportunities for this exciting concept. Someday, in the not too distant future, these boutiques will be in cities and towns around the globe.

To learn how you can bring Women's Health Boutique into your community, call toll free to 888-280-2053. Address your e-mail messages to w-h-bsales@w-h-b.com or send regular mail to Women's Health Boutique, 12715 Telge Road, Cypress, Texas, 77429.

Someone will answer your questions and provide you with all you want to know about this wonderful possibility.

This may well be your legacy to your own mother, and to the legions of women who have suffered in silence because they had no place to turn.

Women's Health Boutique Locations

California
1115 South B Street
San Mateo, CA 94401-4314
650.357.9236
Fax 650.357.9308

Connecticut
420 Post Road West
Westport, CT 06880
203.454.2156
Fax 203.454.0214

Georgia
520 S. Main Street
Alpharetta, GA 30004
770.442.3989
Fax 770.442.9848

1138 E. 72nd Street
Savannah, GA 31404
912.692.0100
Fax 912.692.0107

Ohio
8110 Montgomery Road
Cincinnati, OH 45236
513.936.9098
Fax 513.936.0242

Maryland
15200 Shady Grove Road
Rockville, MD 20850
301.330.1084
Fax 301.330.4167

Michigan
5150 Plainfield, NE
Grand Rapids, MI 49525
616.364.5431
Fax 616.364.4047

26612 Southfield Road
Lathrup Village, MI 48076-4531
248.552.0606
Fax 248.552.0420

New Jersey
441 Main Street
Metuchen, NJ 08840
732.744.1884
Fax 732.744.1887

Oklahoma
12062 North May Avenue
Oklahoma City, OK 73120
405.936.0030
Fax 405.936.0031

Texas
5020 FM 1960 West
Houston, TX 77069
281.895.6954
Fax 281.895.6956

2270/72 West Holcombe
Houston, TX 77030
713.592.6023
Fax 713.592.6029

14048 Memorial Drive
(Memorial & Kirkwood)
Houston, TX 77079
281.531.6582
Fax 281.531.6923

3800-P Spencer Highway
Pasadena, TX 77054
713.947.2099
Fax 713.947.2177

510 E. Loop 281
Longview, TX 75605
903.758.9904
Fax 903.236.9786

WOMEN'S HEALTH BOUTIQUE
31209 Plymouth Rd.
Livonia, MI 48150
(734)762-9324

Author's Resource Material

Breast Cancer
American Cancer Society
National Cancer Institute
Susan G. Komen Breast Cancer Foundation
Mayo Clinic Women's Healthsource, January 1998

Hair Loss
National Cancer Institute
American Hair Loss Council, 1997
National Alopecia Areata Foundation
Susan G. Komen Breast Cancer Foundation

Incontinence
Mayo Clinic Health Letter, January 1998
National Association for Continence (NAFC)
The Bladder Health Council of the
American Foundation for Urologic Disease

Pregnancy and Breastfeeding
Mayo Clinic *Complete Book of Pregnancy & Baby's First Year*
La Leche League International
The Breastfeeding Answer Book
by Nancy Mohrbacher and Julie Stock

General
Smith Barney Research
The New Women's Movement: Women's Healthcare, April 1997

The End

And the Beginning...

*For women everywhere
who will deal with special healthcare issues
at some time in their lives.*

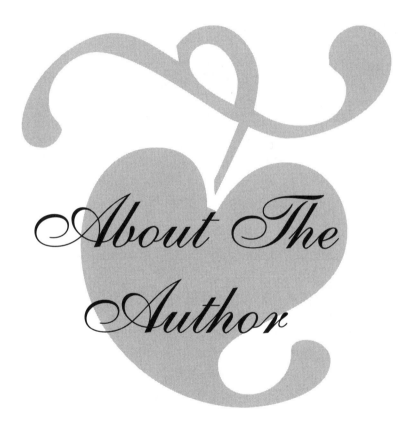

About The Author

*N*ancy Arnold has been writing stuff for other people to read for close to 40 years. She started while in junior high school, handing out the still-wet mimeographed school newspaper containing her reports of school happenings.

As a high school freshman, Nancy was recruited by the Houston Chronicle as a stringer to cover her school's football games every Friday night for the Saturday morning edition. She did this through her high school years, and conducted locker room interviews a decade before women supposedly broke that barrier in professional sports.

Nancy lives in the small town where she grew up, just 30 miles west of Houston. She writes a popular news and events column for the weekly county newspaper, putting a humorous spin on the everyday activities of the community.

For a time, Nancy was news editor of a small weekly newspaper. She was also reporter, photographer and advertising manager. If that wasn't enough, she developed and printed her own photos in a makeshift darkroom. Her children, tired of shouting through the darkroom wall, convinced her to give up the newspaper business and get a "real job."

Nancy writes for the sheer joy of it, and feels it's a God-given talent. An out-going, friendly woman, she views writing as written conversation. Her style has often been described as "word pictures."

Nancy has been associated with the franchise giant ICED since 1979, both on corporate staff and as the owner of a Kwik Kopy Printing franchise in Houston. Through those years, she has been a training instructor for franchisees from around the world, and enjoys many friendships with owners with whom she works. She is also a contributing writer to the international magazine, *Partners,* published by ICED.

Nancy served on the board of Printing Industries of the Gulf

Coast, a trade organization serving the graphic arts industry in Houston and the multi-county surrounding area. She has been a recognized leader in the printing industry, and served as president of the Houston Area Quick Printers for an unprecedented three terms.

In 1994, Nancy received the Outstanding Quick Printer of the Year award, only the third one awarded in a ten-year span. During Nancy's tenure on the HAQPA board, the group began the process of affiliating with the National Association of Quick Printers (NAQP), a task that was completed shortly after Nancy left office.

Nancy considers it a privilege to write the story of Women's Health Boutique. She is grateful, as a woman, to know there's such a place that's just for women. "It's long overdue," says Nancy, "and I'm proud to be part of it."

Heartfelt thanks

*to Pauline Lehmann for her tireless assistance,
reading, re-reading, and offering gentle advice
so this work could move forward.*

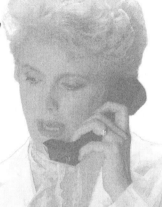

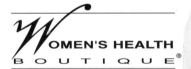